Aphasia Workbook
Foods - Book 2: Fruits & Vegetables

By Florence Jones

This collection of books was created for my father who has Aphasia. Over the months while working with my father on his speech therapy homework, I realized how difficult it was for him to identify the hand-drawn black and white pictures that were presented to him on his worksheets.

In the beginning I remembered the doctor telling me to make every visit a productive visit. Having a tangible book that he can take with him and one that anyone can pick up and use added consistency to his recovery.

I tried workbooks made for children, however, these seemed to insult his intelligence. I also tried computer-based speech therapy applications which were only available when he had access to a computer. He seemed to progress faster when he worked one on one with another human being.

Each page includes photographs of different items common to every day living. Also on each page there are three levels of difficulty. How you choose to use each page is up to you and your patient or loved one. As I worked with my father to help him regain his speech, reading and writing, I realized the process was the same as for a child. First you learn to speak, then read, followed by writing. There are also different levels of Aphasia: one person may regain speaking very quickly while another not so quickly.

Get Started - There are three steps on each page:

Step 1 - Identify the picture: point to the picture and speak it out load. Have your patient or loved one repeat the word over and over, day after day. If your patient or loved one has severe Aphasia you might want to just do this step until your patient or loved one is able to identify the pictures. While working on this section you can reinforce the lesson by using the actual object in the picture.

Step 2 – Use the word in a sentence: this section is designed to help the patient identify the object in use. Each sentence has been chosen to help the patient regain basic sentences for every day use. Read the sentence and fill in the word. Have the patient or loved one try to verbally fill in the word own his own. He or she might need to be cued. While working on this section you can reinforce the lesson by using the actual objects.

Step 3 – Writing: after your patient or loved one has learned the objects the final step is writing the word. Have your patient write over the grayed out word, then encourage him or her to continue on their own.

Apple

1. Point to the picture and say the word. Then have your patient repeat the word.

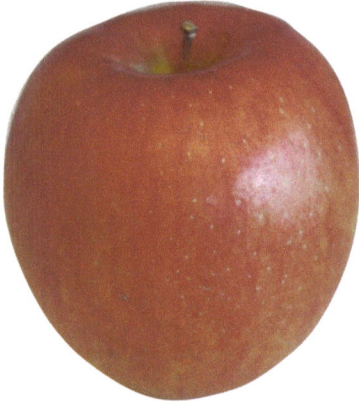

May I have a slice of _____ pie, please.

2. Read the sentence to your patient and verbally fill in the word. Read the sentence again and have your patient verbally fill in the missing word.

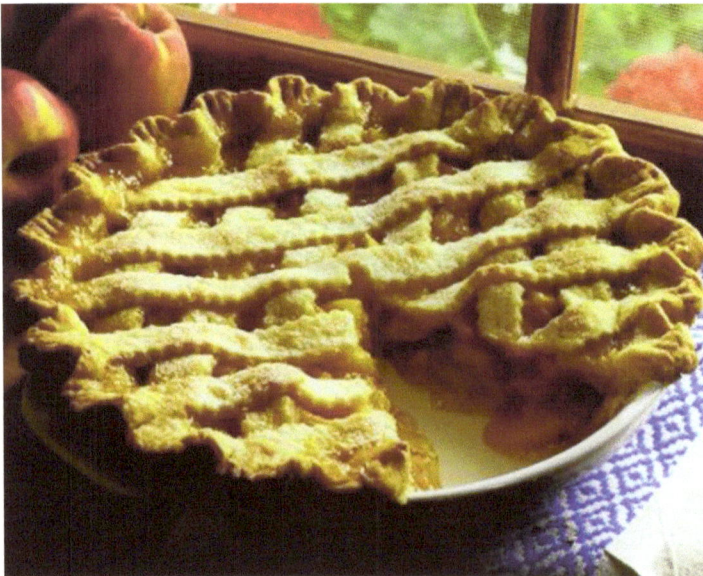

3. Have your patient practice writing the word. Trace over each shaded word then repeat the word several times on each line.

Apple

Apple _____

Apple _____

Apple _____

Apple _____

Apple _____

Apple _____

Apple _____

Apple _____

Apple _____

Apple _____

Apple _____

Apple _____

Apple _____

Apple _____

Apple _____

Bananas

1. Point to the picture and say the word. Then have your patient repeat the word.

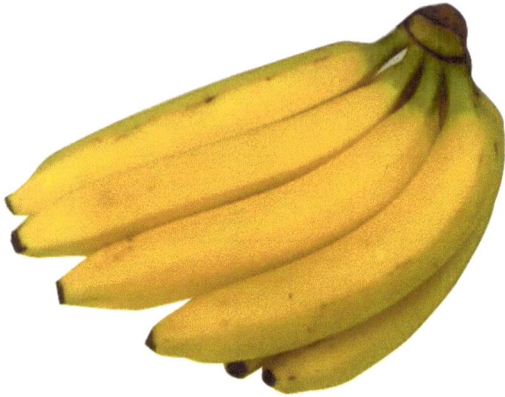

I like _____ on my ceral.

2. Read the sentence to your patient and verbally fill in the word. Read the sentence again and have your patient verbally fill in the missing word.

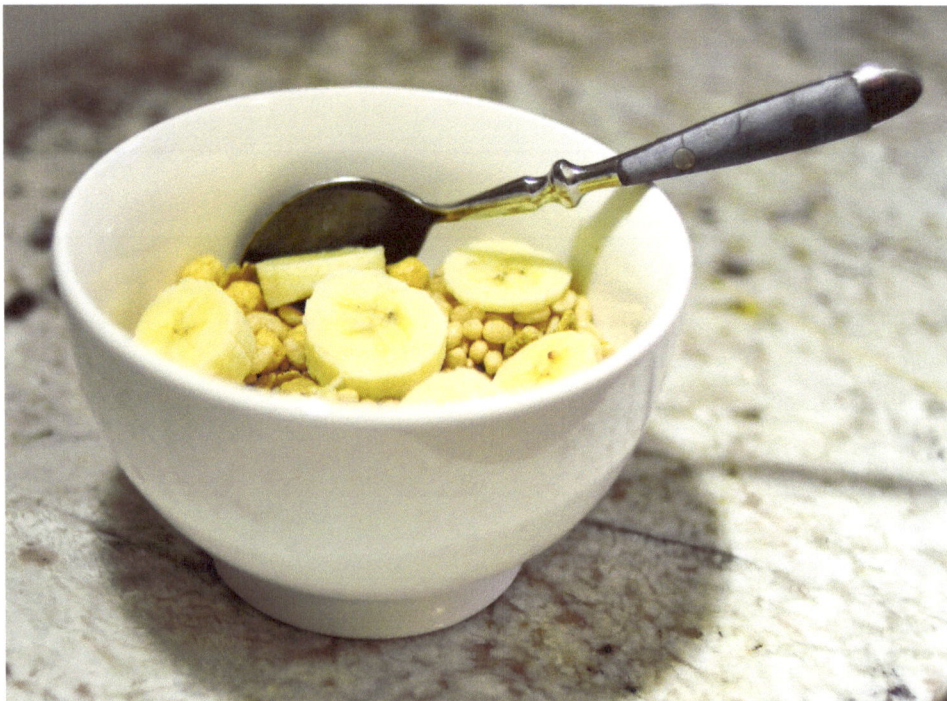

3. Have your patient practice writing the word. Trace over each shaded word then repeat the word several times on each line..

Bananas

Bananas _____

Bananas _____

Bananas _____

Bananas _____

Bananas _____

Bananas _____

Bananas _____

Bananas _____

Bananas _____

Bananas _____

Bananas _____

Bananas _____

Bananas _____

Bananas _____

Bananas _____

Pear

1. Point to the picture and say the word. Then have your patient repeat the word.

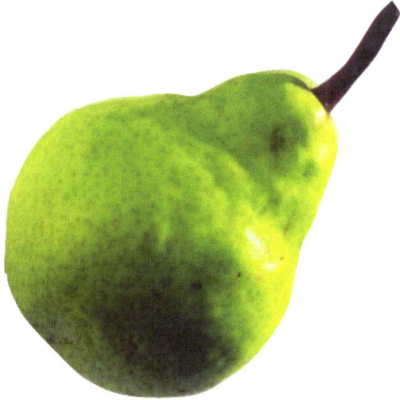

Will you slice my _____ for me, please

2. Read the sentence to your patient and verbally fill in the word. Read the sentence again and have your patient verbally fill in the missing word.

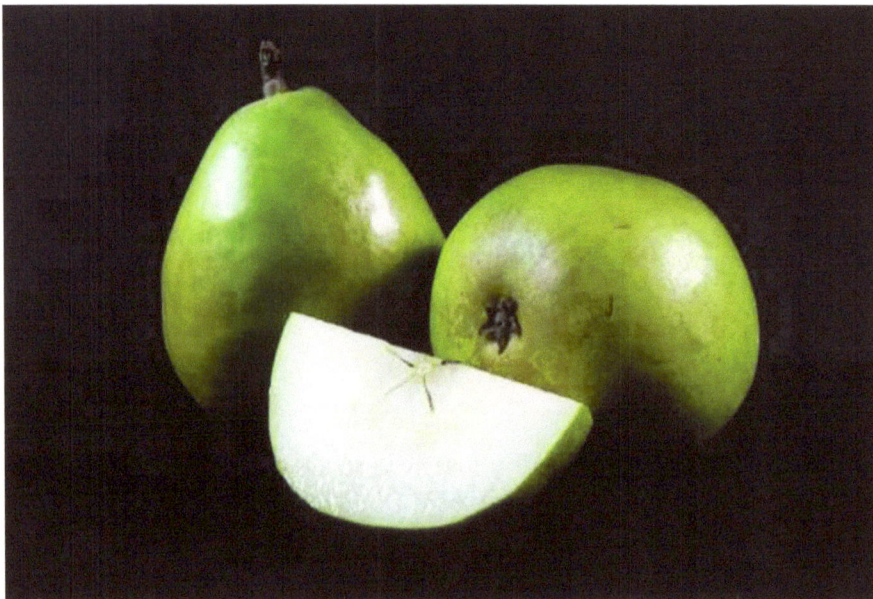

3. Have your patient practice writing the word. Trace over each shaded word then repeat the word several times on each line.

Pear

Pear _____

Pear _____

Pear _____

Pear _____

Pear _____

Pear _____

Pear _____

Pear _____

Pear _____

Pear _____

Pear _____

Pear _____

Pear _____

Pear _____

Pear _____

Tomatoes

1. Point to the picture and say the word. Then have your patient repeat the word.

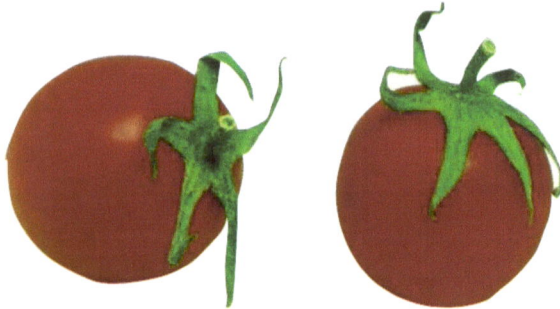

I like _____ in my salad.

2. Read the sentence to your patient and verbally fill in the word. Read the sentence again and have your patient verbally fill in the missing word.

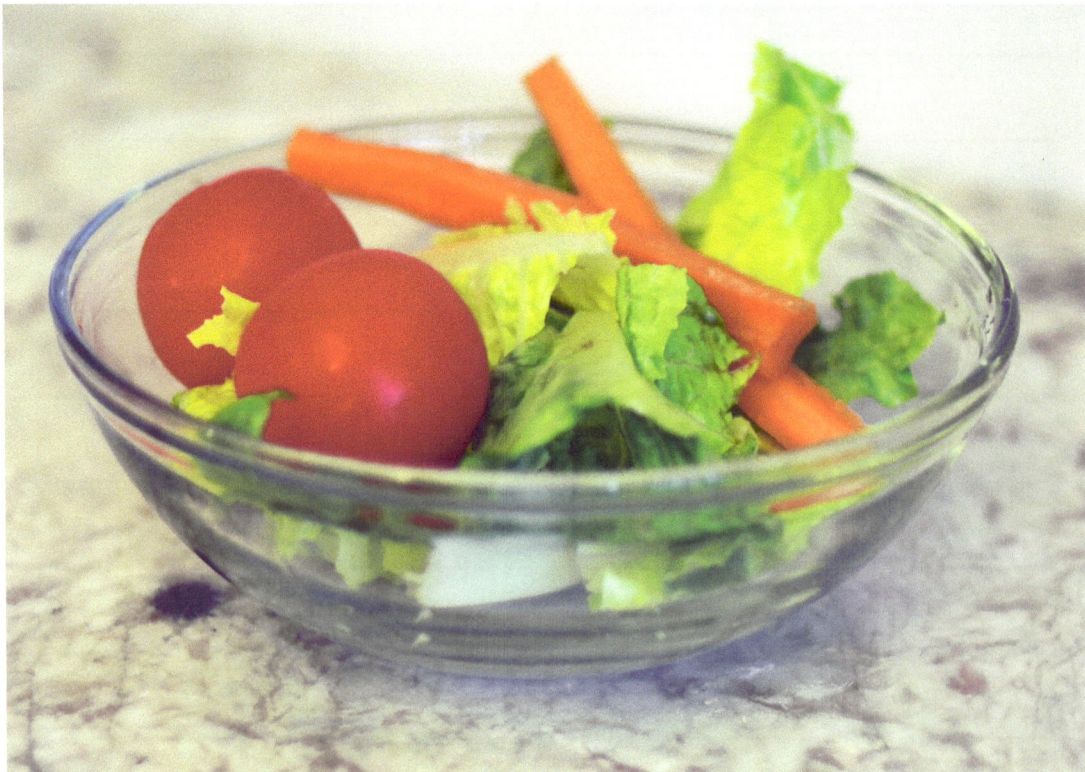

   Aphasia Workbook, Foods - Book 2: Fruits & Vegetables, Copyright 2013

3. Have your patient practice writing the word. Trace over each shaded word then repeat the word several times on each line.

Tomatoes

Tomatoes _____

Tomatoes _____

Tomatoes _____

Tomatoes _____

Tomatoes _____

Tomatoes _____

Tomatoes _____

Tomatoes _____

Tomatoes _____

Tomatoes _____

Tomatoes _____

Tomatoes _____

Tomatoes _____

Tomatoes _____

Tomatoes _____

Lettuce

1. Point to the picture and say the word. Then have your patient repeat the word.

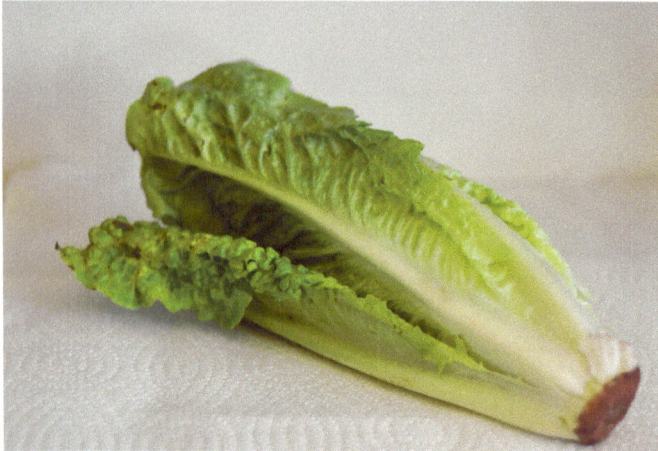

May I have _____ on my burger.

2. Read the sentence to your patient and verbally fill in the word. Read the sentence again and have your patient verbally fill in the missing word.

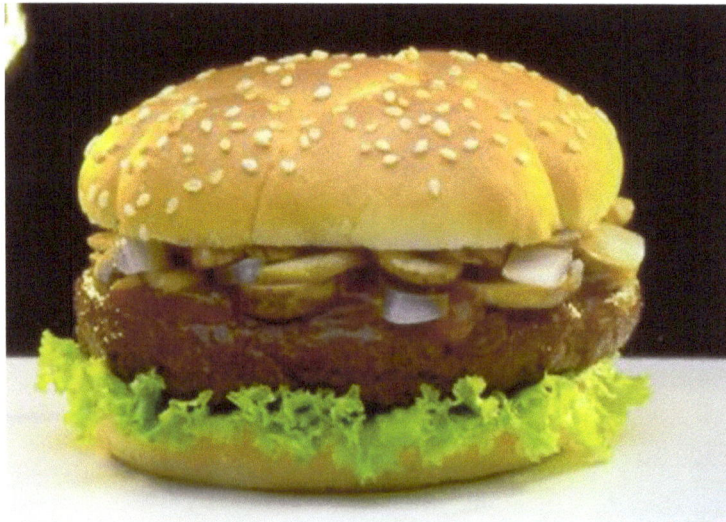

3. Have your patient practice writing the word. Trace over each shaded word then repeat the word several times on each line.

Lettuce

Lettuce _____

Lettuce _____

Lettuce _____

Lettuce _____

Lettuce _____

Lettuce _____

Lettuce _____

Lettuce _____

Lettuce _____

Lettuce _____

Lettuce _____

Lettuce _____

Lettuce _____

Lettuce _____

Lettuce _____

Carrot

1. Point to the picture and say the word. Then have your patient repeat the word.

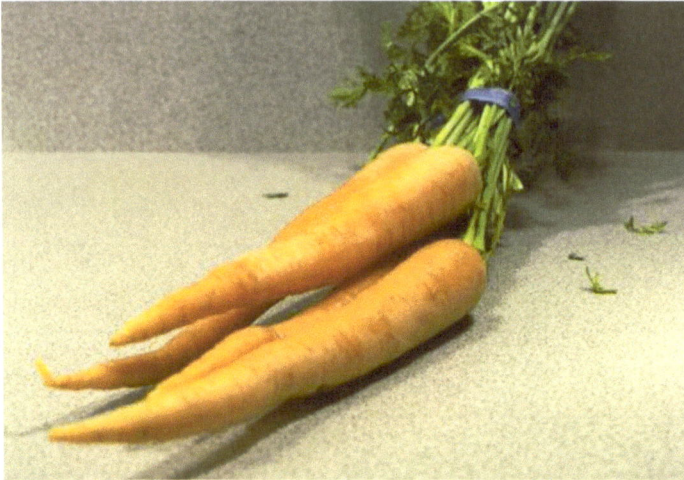

I need to peel the _____.

2. Read the sentence to your patient and verbally fill in the word. Read the sentence again and have your patient verbally fill in the missing word.

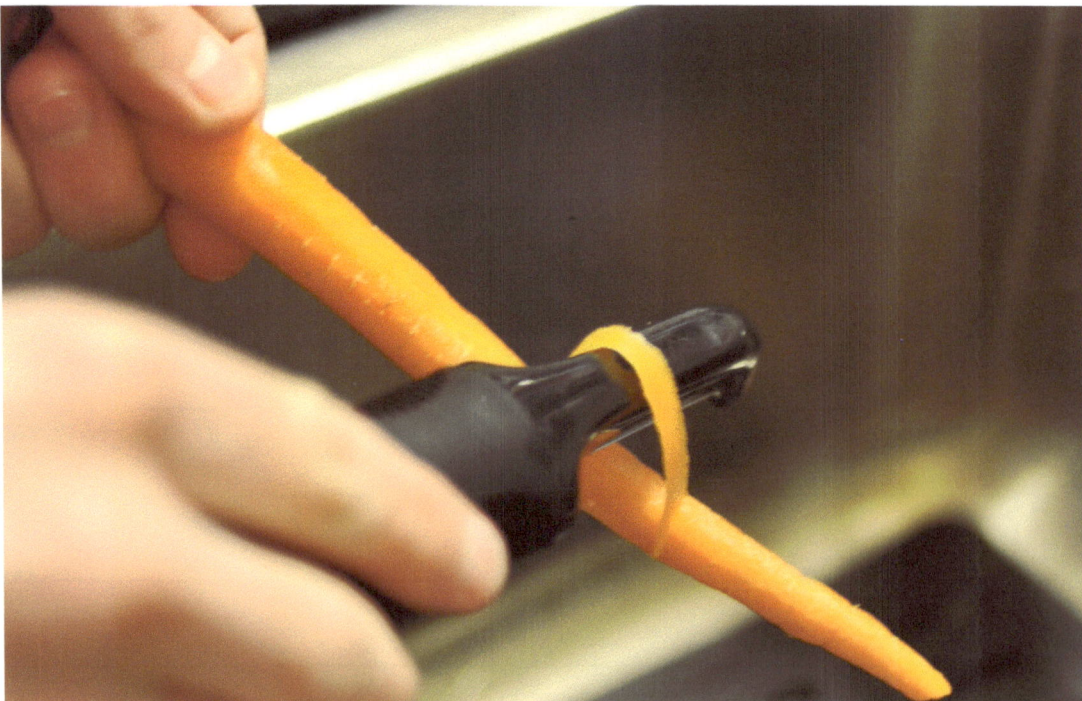

3. Have your patient practice writing the word. Trace over each shaded word then repeat the word several times on each line.

Carrot

Carrot _____

Carrot _____

Carrot _____

Carrot _____

Carrot _____

Carrot _____

Carrot _____

Carrot _____

Carrot _____

Carrot _____

Carrot _____

Carrot _____

Carrot _____

Carrot _____

Carrot _____

Carrot _____

Grapes

1. Point to the picture and say the word. Then have your patient repeat the word.

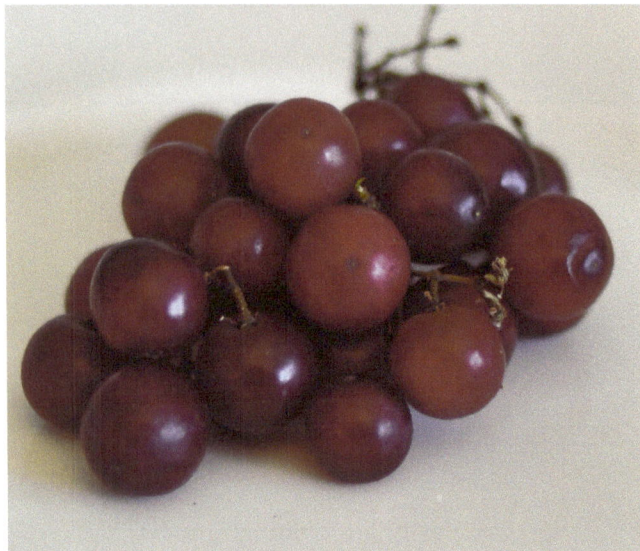

I like _____ with wine and cheese.

2. Read the sentence to your patient and verbally fill in the word. Read the sentence again and have your patient verbally fill in the missing word.

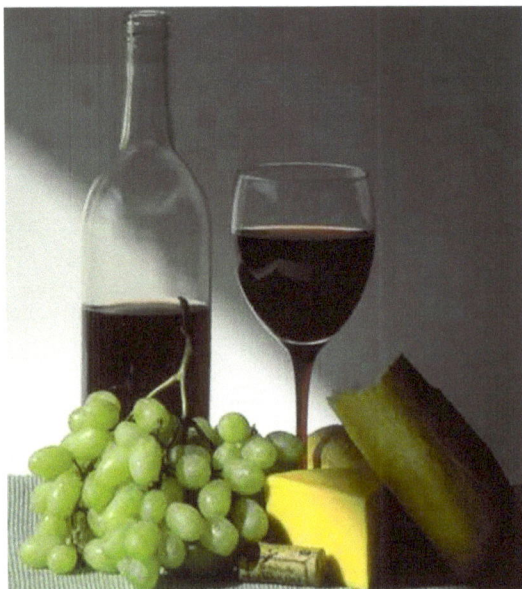

3. Have your patient practice writing the word. Trace over each shaded word then repeat the word several times on each line.

Grapes

Grapes _____

Grapes _____

Grapes _____

Grapes _____

Grapes _____

Grapes _____

Grapes _____

Grapes _____

Grapes _____

Grapes _____

Grapes _____

Grapes _____

Grapes _____

Grapes _____

Grapes _____

Grapes _____

Strawberry

1. Point to the picture and say the word. Then have your patient repeat the word.

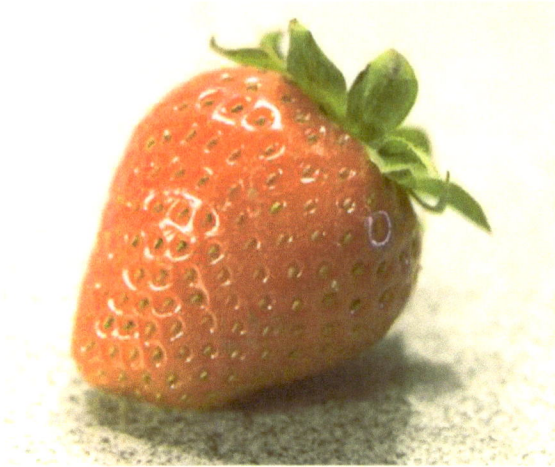

I love _____ tipped in chocolate.

2. Read the sentence to your patient and verbally fill in the word. Read the sentence again and have your patient verbally fill in the missing word.

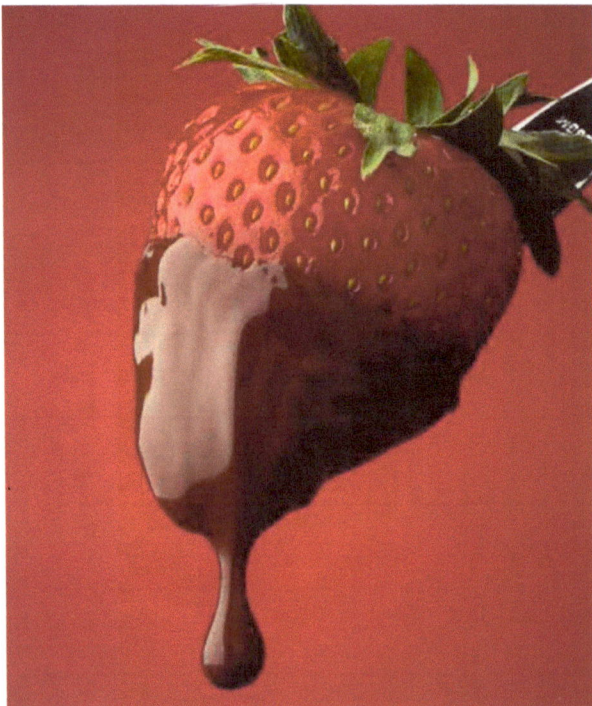

3. Have your patient practice writing the word. Trace over each shaded word then repeat the word several times on each line.

Strawberry

Strawberry _____

Strawberry _____

Strawberry _____

Strawberry _____

Strawberry _____

Strawberry _____

Strawberry _____

Strawberry _____

Strawberry _____

Strawberry _____

Strawberry _____

Strawberry _____

Strawberry _____

Strawberry _____

Strawberry _____

Strawberry _____

Asparagus

1. Point to the picture and say the word. Then have your patient repeat the word.

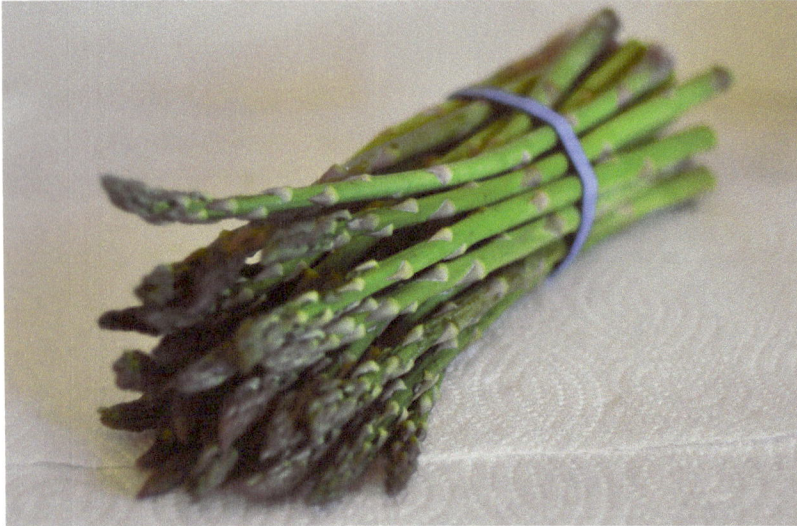

I like _____with dinner.

2. Read the sentence to your patient and verbally fill in the word. Read the sentence again and have your patient verbally fill in the missing word.

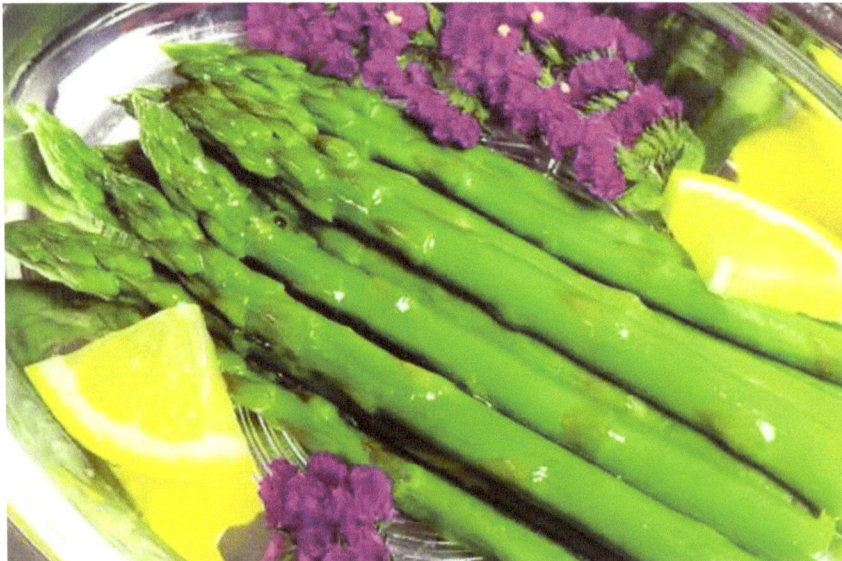

Aphasia Workbook, Foods - Book 2: Fruits & Vegetables, Copyright 2013

3. Have your patient practice writing the word. Trace over each shaded word then repeat the word several times on each line.

Asparagus

Asparagus _____

Asparagus _____

Asparagus _____

Asparagus _____

Asparagus _____

Asparagus _____

Asparagus _____

Asparagus _____

Asparagus _____

Asparagus _____

Asparagus _____

Asparagus _____

Asparagus _____

Asparagus _____

Asparagus _____

Asparagus _____

Pineapple

1. Point to the picture and say the word. Then have your patient repeat the word.

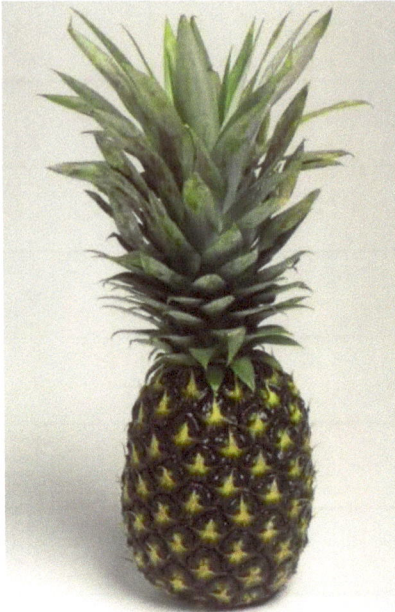

Would you open the can of _____ for me. please.

2. Read the sentence to your patient and verbally fill in the word. Read the sentence again and have your patient verbally fill in the missing word.

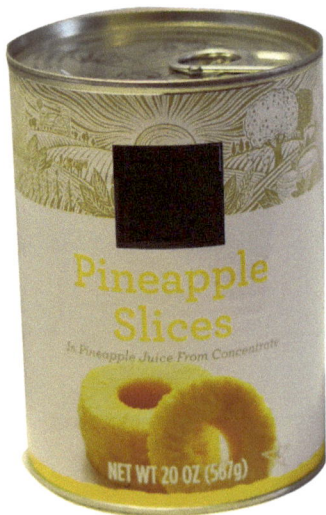

Aphasia Workbook, Foods - Book 2: Fruits & Vegetables, Copyright 2013

3. Have your patient practice writing the word. Trace over each shaded word then repeat the word several times on each line.

Pineapple

Pineapple _____

Pineapple _____

Pineapple _____

Pineapple _____

Pineapple _____

Pineapple _____

Pineapple _____

Pineapple _____

Pineapple _____

Pineapple _____

Pineapple _____

Pineapple _____

Pineapple _____

Pineapple _____

Pineapple _____

Pineapple _____

Pepper

1. Point to the picture and say the word. Then have your patient repeat the word.

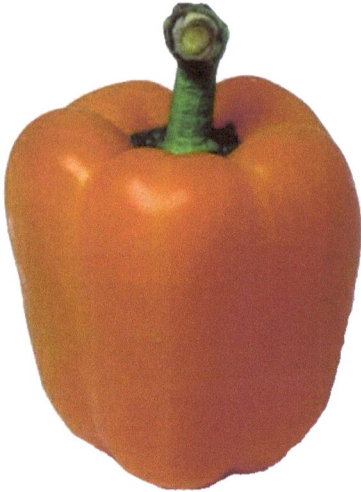

A like all _____(s), green, red or yellow.

2. Read the sentence to your patient and verbally fill in the word. Read the sentence again and have your patient verbally fill in the missing word.

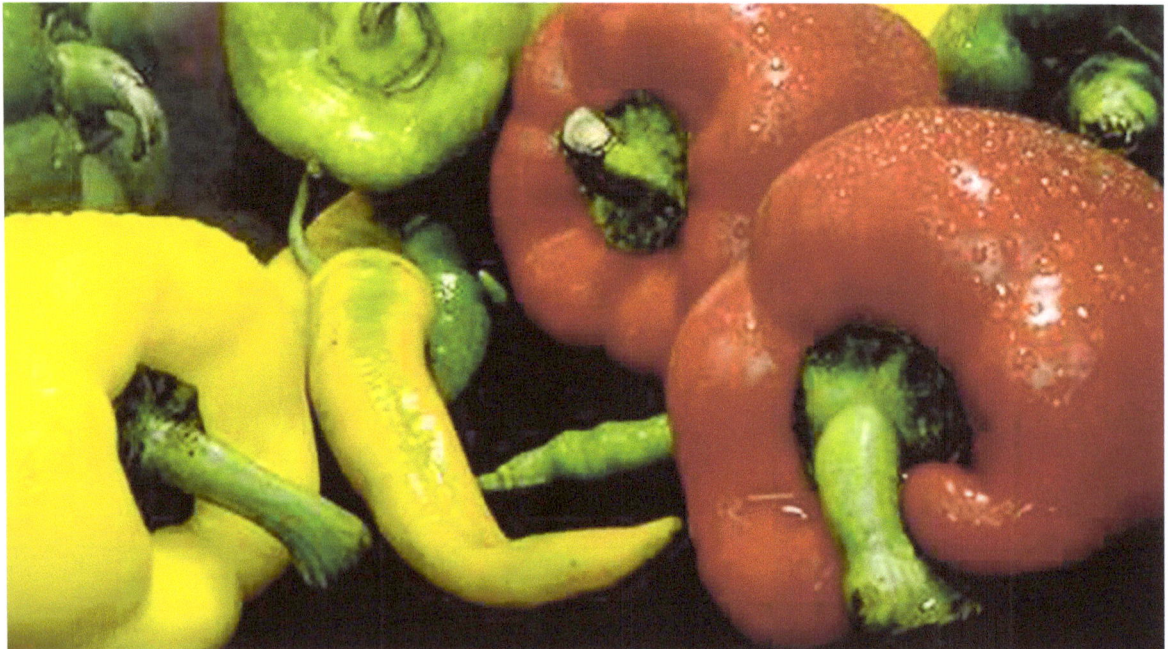

3. Have your patient practice writing the word. Trace over each shaded word then repeat the word several times on each line.

Pepper

Pepper _____

Pepper _____

Pepper _____

Pepper _____

Pepper _____

Pepper _____

Pepper _____

Pepper _____

Pepper _____

Pepper _____

Pepper _____

Pepper _____

Pepper _____

Pepper _____

Pepper _____

Orange

1. Point to the picture and say the word. Then have your patient repeat the word.

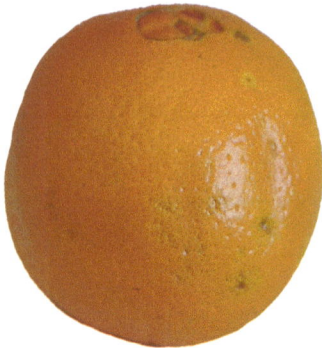

I like _____ juice for breakfast.

2. Read the sentence to your patient and verbally fill in the word. Read the sentence again and have your patient verbally fill in the missing word.

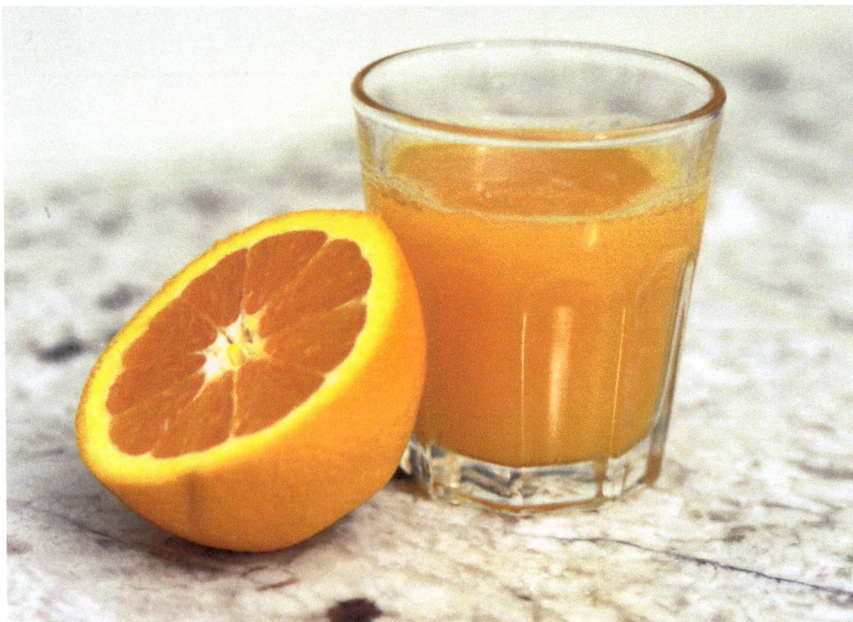

3. Have your patient practice writing the word. Trace over each shaded word then repeat the word several times on each line.

Orange

Orange _____

Orange _____

Orange _____

Orange _____

Orange _____

Orange _____

Orange _____

Orange _____

Orange _____

Orange _____

Orange _____

Orange _____

Orange _____

Orange _____

Orange _____

Broccoli

1. Point to the picture and say the word. Then have your patient repeat the word.

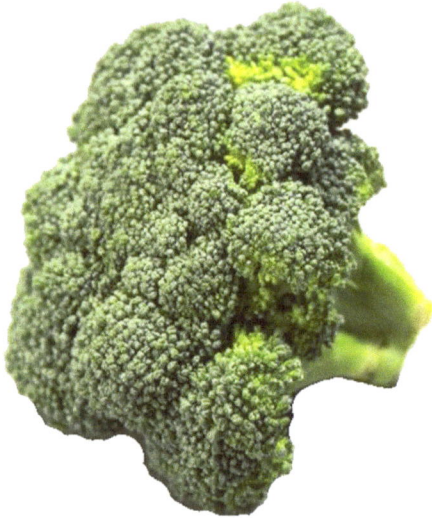

May I have _____ for dinner, please.

2. Read the sentence to your patient and verbally fill in the word. Read the sentence again and have your patient verbally fill in the missing word.

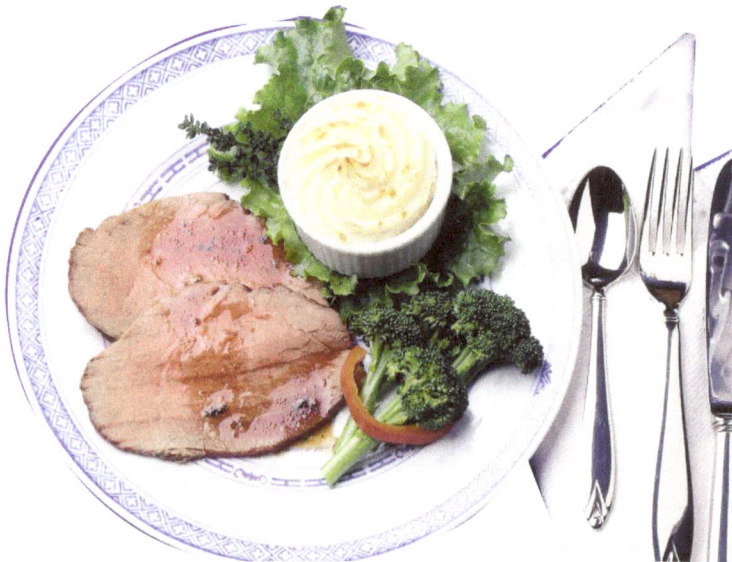

3. Have your patient practice writing the word. Trace over each shaded word then repeat the word several times on each line.

Broccoli

Broccoli_____

Broccoli_____

Broccoli_____

Broccoli_____

Broccoli_____

Broccoli_____

Broccoli_____

Broccoli_____

Broccoli_____

Broccoli_____

Broccoli_____

Broccoli_____

Broccoli_____

Broccoli_____

Broccoli_____

Blueberries

1. Point to the picture and say the word. Then have your patient repeat the word.

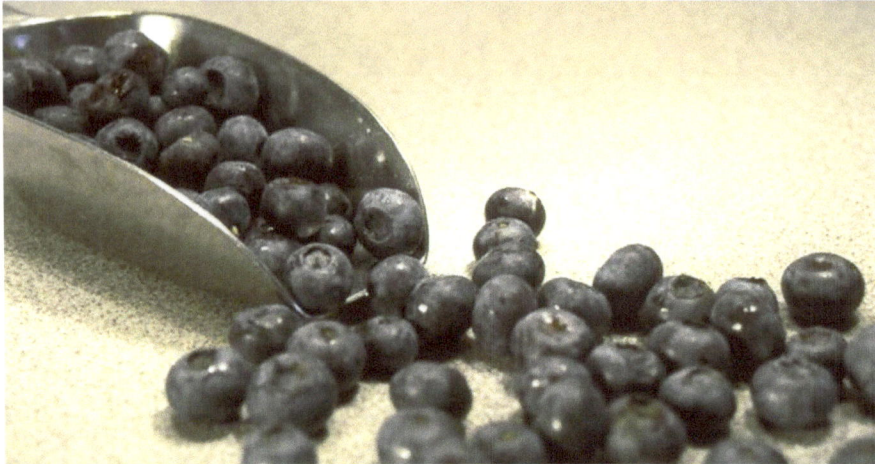

I like _____ on my ceral.

2. Read the sentence to your patient and verbally fill in the word. Read the sentence again and have your patient verbally fill in the missing word.

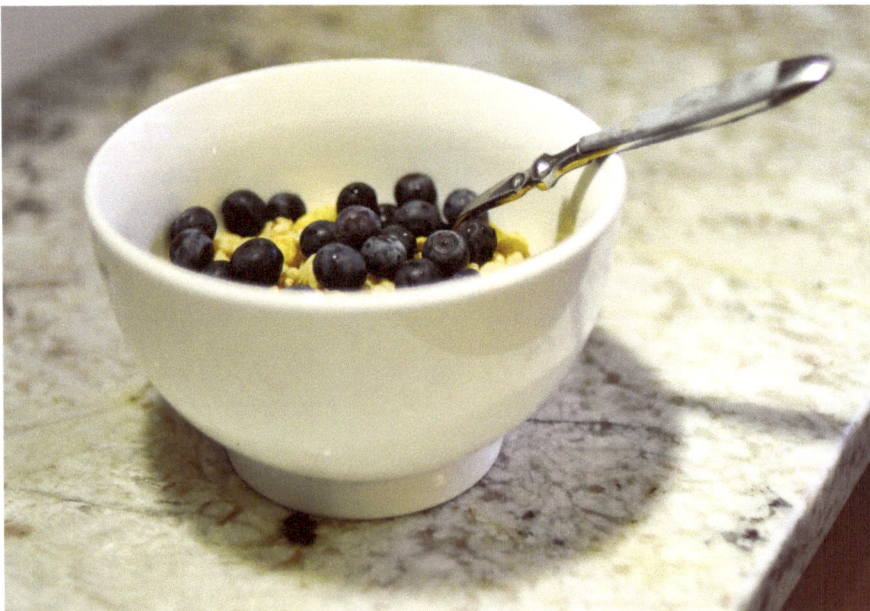

3. Have your patient practice writing the word. Trace over each shaded word then repeat the word several times on each line.

Blueberries

Blueberries _____

Blueberries _____

Blueberries _____

Blueberries _____

Blueberries _____

Blueberries _____

Blueberries _____

Blueberries _____

Blueberries _____

Blueberries _____

Blueberries _____

Blueberries _____

Blueberries _____

Blueberries _____

Blueberries _____

Blueberries _____

Peas

1. Point to the picture and say the word. Then have your patient repeat the word.

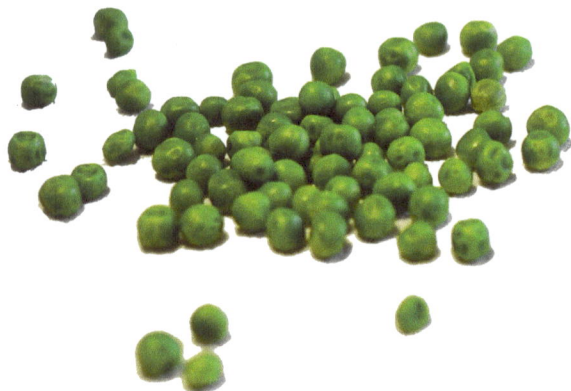

May I have _____ for dinner, please.

2. Read the sentence to your patient and verbally fill in the word. Read the sentence again and have your patient verbally fill in the missing word.

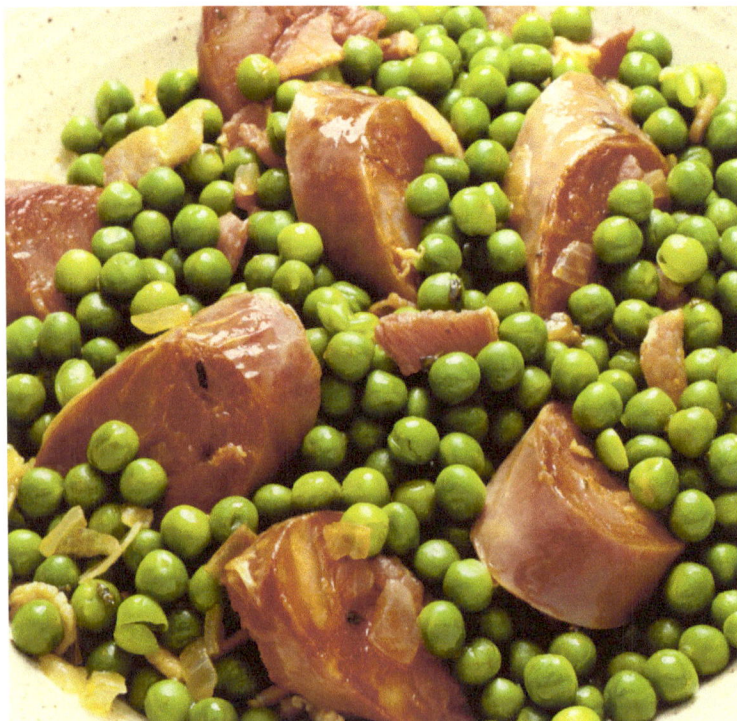

3. Have your patient practice writing the word. Trace over each shaded word then repeat the word several times on each line.

Peas

Peas _____

Peas _____

Peas _____

Peas _____

Peas _____

Peas _____

Peas _____

Peas _____

Peas _____

Peas _____

Peas _____

Peas _____

Peas _____

Peas _____

Peas _____

String Beans

1. Point to the picture and say the word. Then have your patient repeat the word.

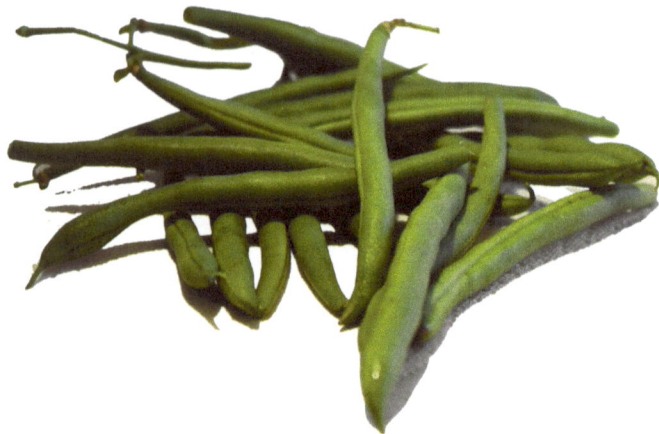

May I have _____for dinner, please.

2. Read the sentence to your patient and verbally fill in the word. Read the sentence again and have your patient verbally fill in the missing word.

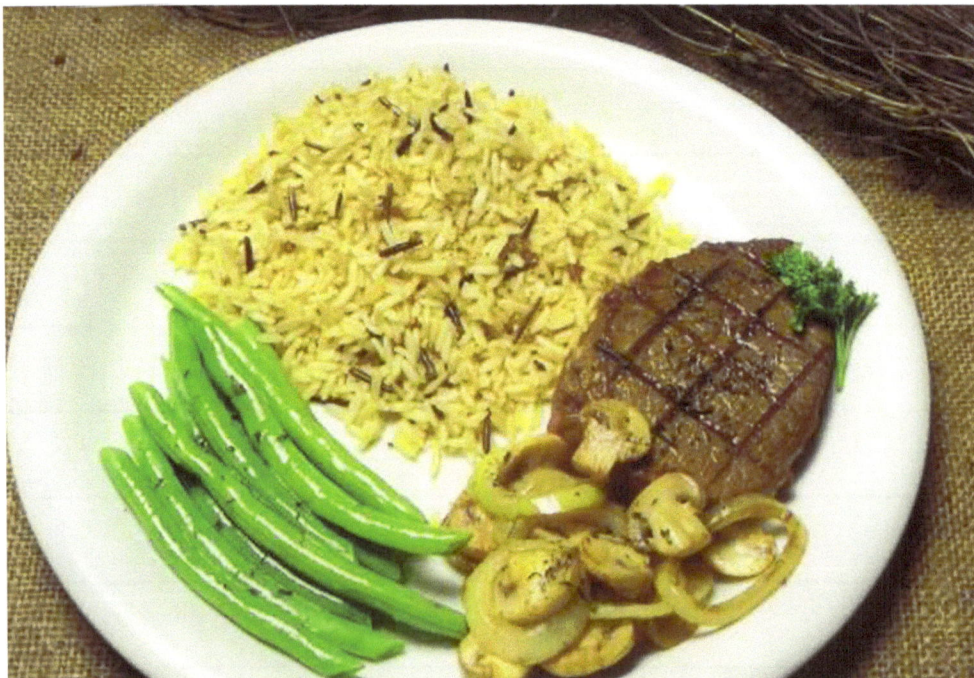

Aphasia Workbook, Foods - Book 2: Fruits & Vegetables, Copyright 2013

3. Have your patient practice writing the word. Trace over each shaded word then repeat the word several times on each line.

String Beans

String Beans _____

String Beans _____

String Beans _____

String Beans _____

String Beans _____

String Beans _____

String Beans _____

String Beans _____

String Beans _____

String Beans _____

String Beans _____

String Beans _____

String Beans _____

String Beans _____

String Beans _____

Cucumber

1. Point to the picture and say the word. Then have your patient repeat the word.

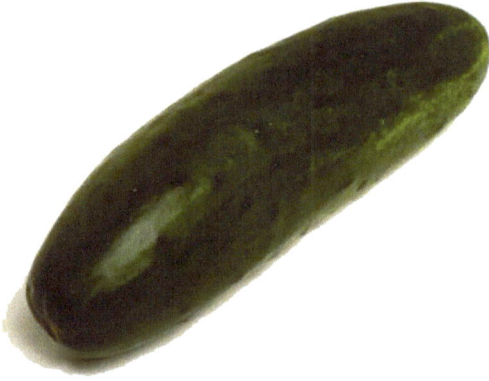

Would you slice my _____, please.

2. Read the sentence to your patient and verbally fill in the word. Read the sentence again and have your patient verbally fill in the missing word.

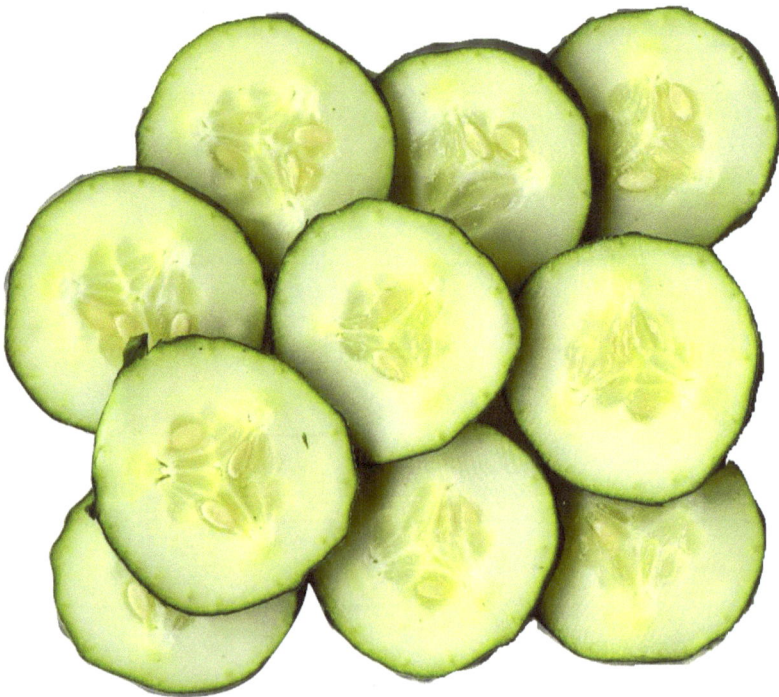

Aphasia Workbook, Foods - Book 2: Fruits & Vegetables, Copyright 2013

3. Have your patient practice writing the word. Trace over each shaded word then repeat the word several times on each line.

Cucumber

Cucumber _____

Cucumber _____

Cucumber _____

Cucumber _____

Cucumber _____

Cucumber _____

Cucumber _____

Cucumber _____

Cucumber _____

Cucumber _____

Cucumber _____

Cucumber _____

Cucumber _____

Cucumber _____

Cucumber _____

Cucumber _____

Potato

1. Point to the picture and say the word. Then have your patient repeat the word.

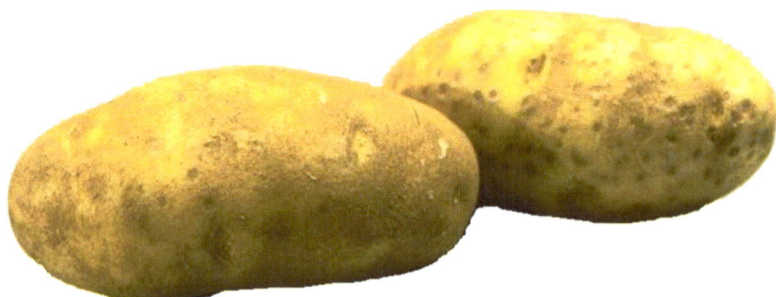

I like a baked_____ with sour cream.

2. Read the sentence to your patient and verbally fill in the word. Read the sentence again and have your patient verbally fill in the missing word.

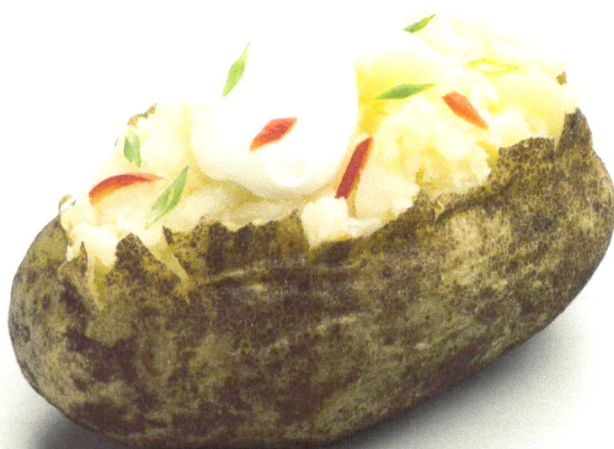

Aphasia Workbook, Foods - Book 2: Fruits & Vegetables, Copyright 2013

3. Have your patient practice writing the word. Trace over each shaded word then repeat the word several times on each line.

Potato

Potato _____

Potato _____

Potato _____

Potato _____

Potato _____

Potato _____

Potato _____

Potato _____

PPotato _____

Potato _____

Potato _____

Potato _____

Potato _____

Potato _____

Potato _____

Potato _____

Kiwi

1. Point to the picture and say the word. Then have your patient repeat the word.

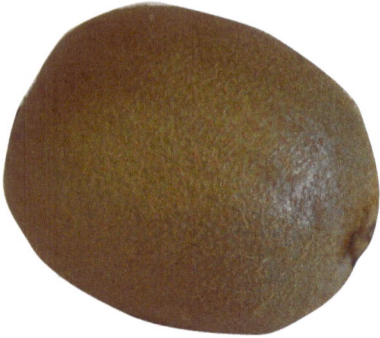

I like a _____for a snack.

2. Read the sentence to your patient and verbally fill in the word. Read the sentence again and have your patient verbally fill in the missing word.

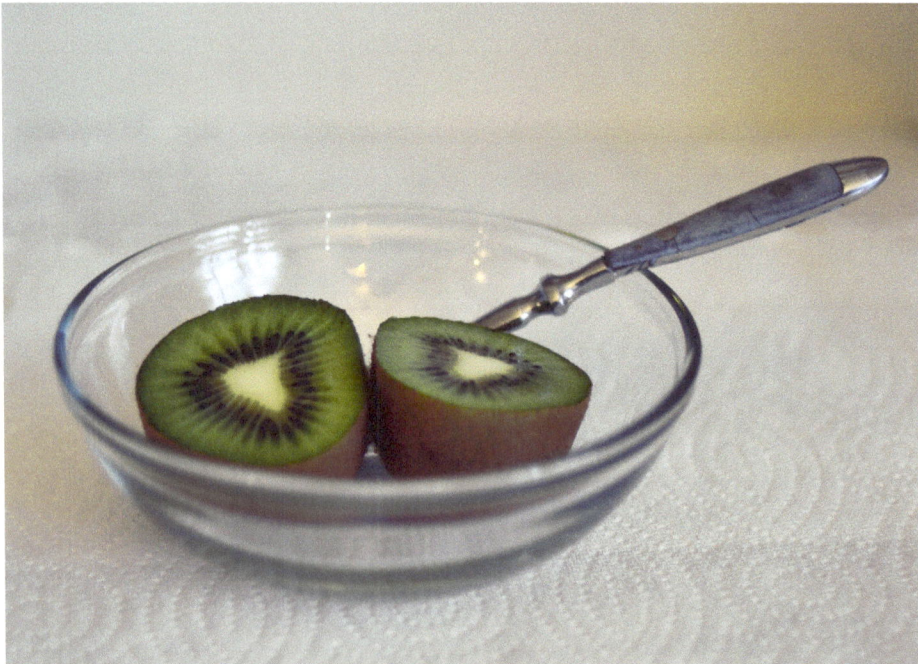

3. Have your patient practice writing the word. Trace over each shaded word then repeat the word several times on each line.

Kiwi

Kiwi _____

Kiwi _____

Kiwi _____

Kiwi _____

Kiwi _____

Kiwi _____

Kiwi _____

Kiwi _____

Kiwi _____

Kiwi _____

Kiwi _____

Kiwi _____

Kiwi _____

Kiwi _____

Kiwi _____

Peaches

1. Point to the picture and say the word. Then have your patient repeat the word.

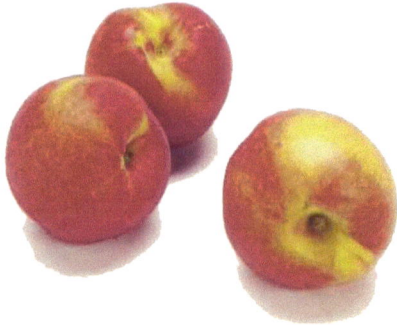

I like cream on my _____.

2. Read the sentence to your patient and verbally fill in the word. Read the sentence again and have your patient verbally fill in the missing word.

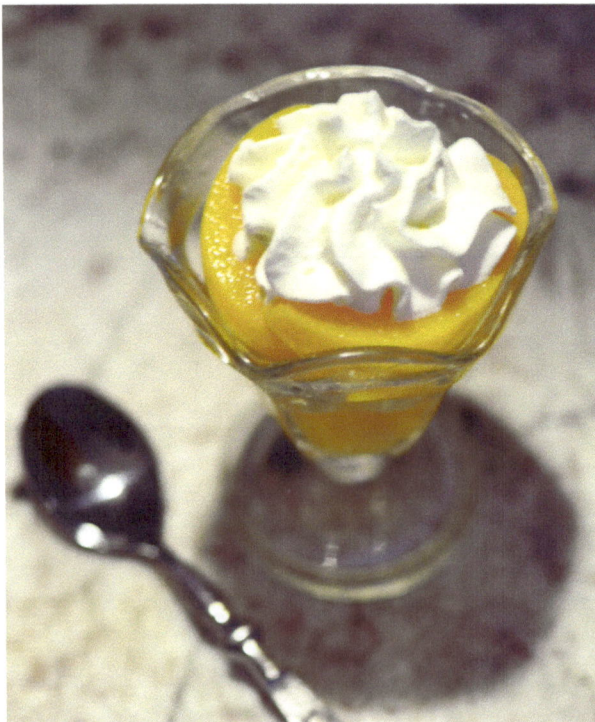

3. Have your patient practice writing the word. Trace over each shaded word then repeat the word several times on each line.

Peaches

Peaches _____

Peaches _____

Peaches _____

Peaches _____

Peaches _____

Peaches _____

Peaches _____

Peaches _____

Peaches _____

Peaches _____

Peaches _____

Peaches _____

Peaches _____

Peaches _____

Peaches _____

Peaches _____

Cherries

1. Point to the picture and say the word. Then have your patient repeat the word.

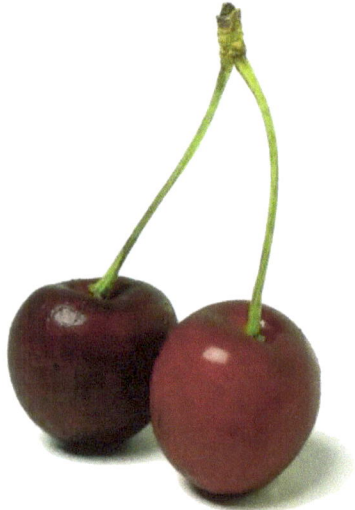

May I have _____ pie for a snack, please.

2. Read the sentence to your patient and verbally fill in the word. Read the sentence again and have your patient verbally fill in the missing word.

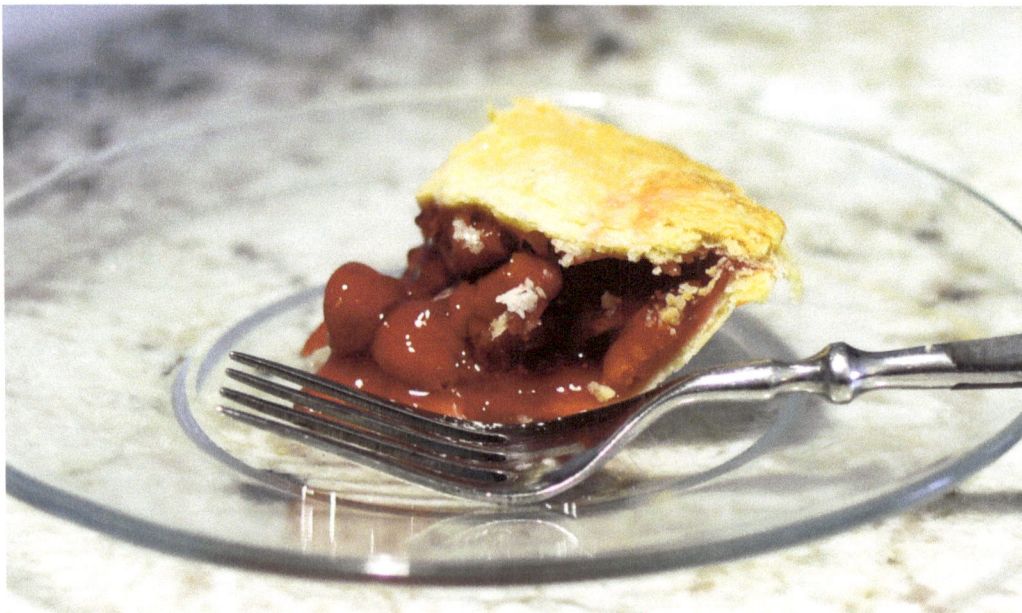

Aphasia Workbook, Foods - Book 2: Fruits & Vegetables, Copyright 2013

3. Have your patient practice writing the word. Trace over each shaded word then repeat the word several times on each line.

Cherries

Cherries _____

Cherries _____

Cherries _____

Cherries _____

Cherries _____

Cherries _____

Cherries _____

Cherries _____

Cherries _____

Cherries _____

Cherries _____

Cherries _____

Cherries _____

Cherries _____

Cherries _____

Cherries _____

Lemon

1. Point to the picture and say the word. Then have your patient repeat the word.

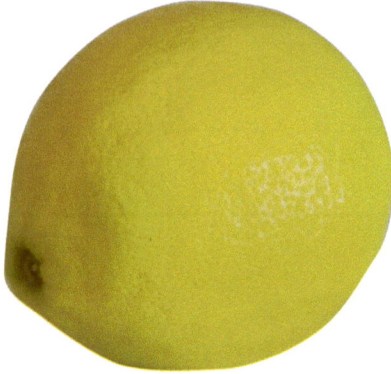

I Like _____ in my tea.

2. Read the sentence to your patient and verbally fill in the word. Read the sentence again and have your patient verbally fill in the missing word.

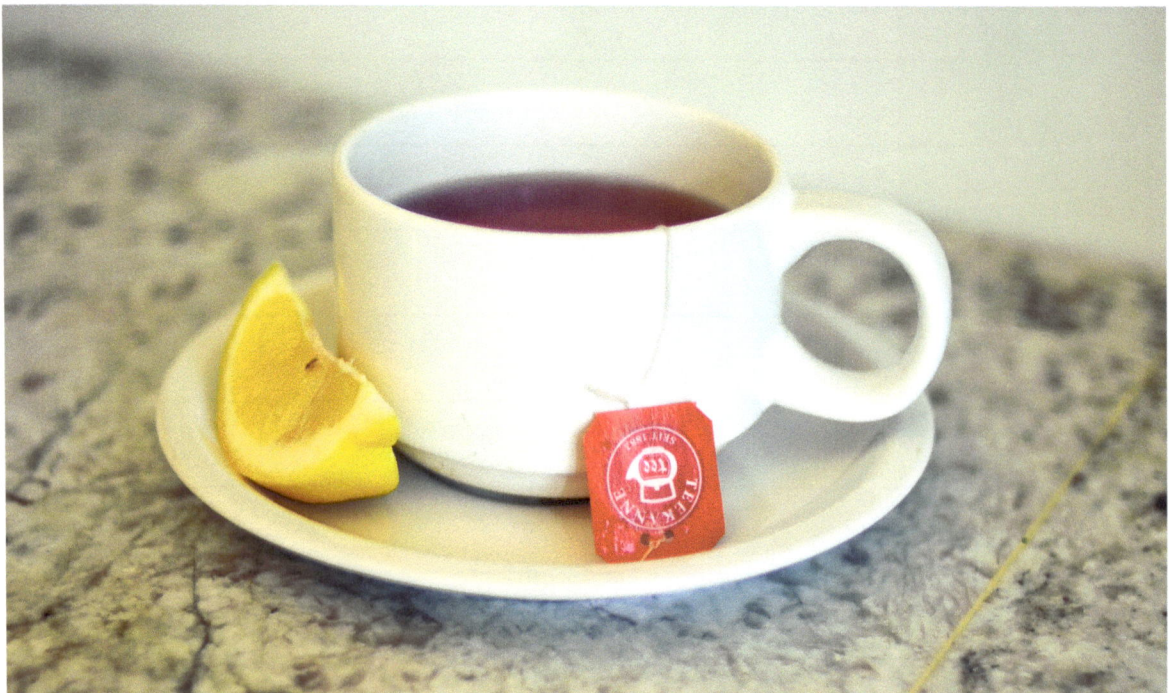

3. Have your patient practice writing the word. Trace over each shaded word then repeat the word several times on each line.

Lemon

Lemon _____

Lemon _____

Lemon _____

Lemon _____

Lemon _____

Lemon _____

Lemon _____

Lemon _____

Lemon _____

Lemon _____

Lemon _____

Lemon _____

Lemon _____

Lemon _____

Lemon _____

Melon

1. Point to the picture and say the word. Then have your patient repeat the word.

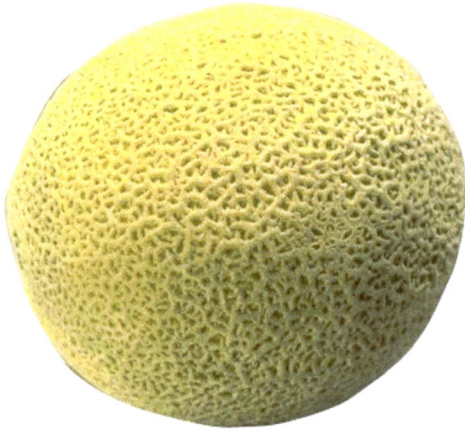

May I have a slice of _____, please.

2. Read the sentence to your patient and verbally fill in the word. Read the sentence again and have your patient verbally fill in the missing word.

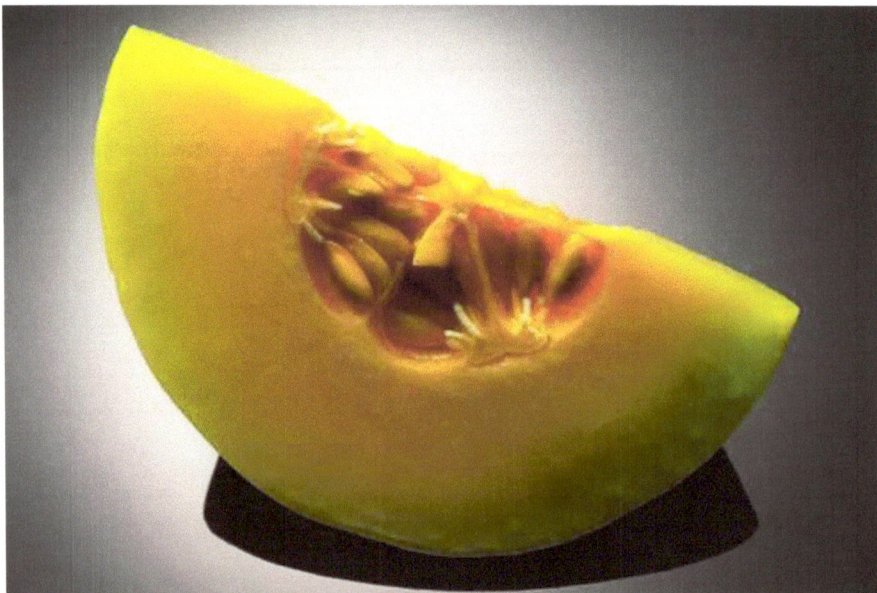

3. Have your patient practice writing the word. Trace over each shaded word then repeat the word several times on each line.

Melon

Melon _____

Melon _____

Melon _____

Melon _____

Melon _____

Melon _____

Melon _____

Melon _____

Melon _____

Melon _____

Melon _____

Melon _____

Melon _____

Melon _____

Melon _____

Melon _____

www.ingramcontent.com/pod-product-compliance
Lightning Source LLC
Chambersburg PA
CBHW060818270326
41930CB00002B/75